Endorsements for
"Darwin's Replacement" (First Edition)

"The need for a superintelligent force to create and sustain living things is well set out and without question. I also appreciated all the research that was done to demonstrate the historical importance and recognition of God in the nation lives of the four nations you selected." -- George Matzko, PhD

"*Darwin's Replacement* is a well-written review of the enormous complexity of all life from the perspective of the molecular foundation. The complexity is more than amazing. Most people enjoy learning about amazing feats, and thus the popularity of 'Ripley's Believe It or Not' and similar books. Our body and its complexity is familiar to all and works so well for most of us that we often take it for granted. Mr. Rogers' book helps us to realize that we are all walking miracles and understanding how it functions is both awe-inspiring and helps us to appreciate the body we all live in while on this earth."
-- Jerry Bergman, PhD

"*Darwin's Replacement* provides a credible assessment of the weaknesses within mainstream evolution theory and proposes a reasonable, evidence-based alternative for the origin and development of life." -- Nicholas Comninellis, MD MPH

"ATOMIC BIOLOGY promises to restore the true foundations of science back to the realm of observation. Current forays into metaphysical speculation and presupposition by 'experts' seem to have caused division, confusion, and misunderstanding in the scientific conversation." -- Jack Taylor, PhD

"My recommendation would be to rework the book as a series of 1-2 page studies for adult Sunday school classes and/or Christian High School classes. It could be useful as an introduction to the topics, in that format." -- David Snoke, PhD

"Your book demonstrates the amazing complexity of life, starting with even the simplest cell, and the numerous conditions needed to sustain life. That all this could be the result of blind, random evolution is highly implausible, and statistically virtually impossible. Hence, as your book concludes, this points to a superintelligent Creator. Your book also notes that the USA, the UK, Canada, and Australia were all founded on submission to the Christian God, and urges those countries return to acknowledging God, also in science classrooms.

I heartily agree with all this." -- John Byl, PhD

"There are only two possibilities for the existence of life: accidental or purposeful. Using science and mathematics, Atomic Biology proves beyond a shadow of doubt that life cannot be accidental. Then the book shows that the only being capable of the creation of life and its orchestrated maintenance is the historical Omniscient, Omnipotent, and Omnipresent Triune God of the Bible and our Nation." -- Sharon Cargo, DVM

"Hi, (LRG): I recently bought the book and am reading it slowly and out loud to myself so that it sticks, but can I say that when I heard Mr. Rogers on Vision I knew that this was a book I'd been waiting for a very long time. I honestly can't put into words how exciting this is for me to finally have something I can refer to when discussing creation and not sound like a loony." -- Linda Houston, Australia

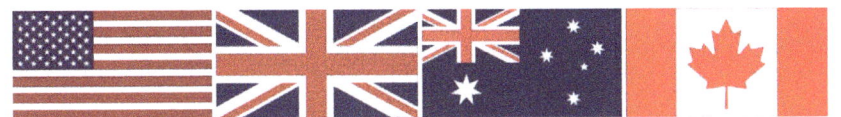

Flags of Four of the Nations Where God Is Part of Government   *

DARWIN'S REPLACEMENT SERIES - FOR EVERYONE

GOD'S GIVEN REASONS
FOR GRATITUDE, PRAISE, AND JOY

JERRY BERGMAN - GRAHAM McLENNAN – THOMAS ROGERS

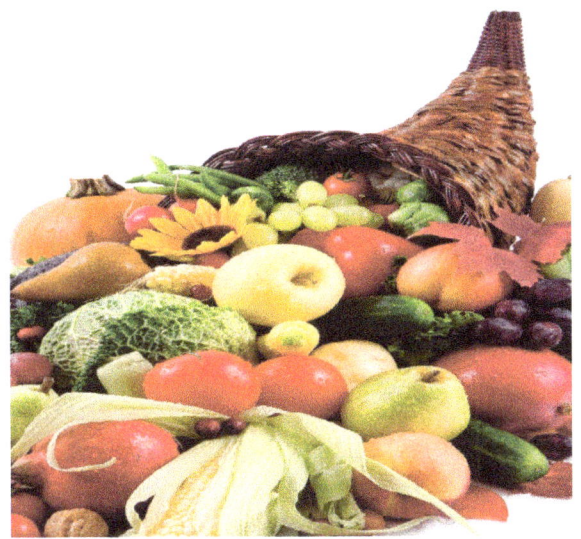

Olga Lyubkina/Shutterstock.com

How are we so amazingly made and cared for? Research now shows us that it requires a superintelligent, reliable, and caring creator. Our Governments and the majority of our citizens call this creator, "God." He makes us from the "dust" using His awesome two-step process: (1) selecting the correct atoms from the soil to create our grown foods, then (2) selecting the correct atoms from our foods to create our cell parts and us.

Who else can make our grown foods and us out of "dust"?

By definition, Darwin's evolution has no intelligence to use.

*Shutterstock Flags: US & UK - Claudio Divisia; Aus.- Artgraphixel; Can. – Jannoon028

DARWIN'S REPLACEMENT SERIES – FOR EVERYONE

GOD'S GIVEN REASONS
FOR GRATITUDE, PRAISE, AND JOY

Part of "THE TRUTH FOR LIFE EDUCATION PROJECT"

LRG

LIFETIME REFERENCE GUIDES INC.
P.O.Box 51613 RPO Park Royal
West Vancouver, BC, Canada   V7T 2X9

www.lifetimereferenceguides.com

www.GodsBiology.com

Copyright © 2025 by Lifetime Reference Guides Inc.

Cover design by ArneeonMedia.com with Shutterstock images: Hands by Chairoij, Fetus by SciePro, Vitruvian Man by Janaka Dharmasena, plus Atom by Arneeon, and Apple by Twenty20Photos/Envato.

All rights reserved.

No part of this publication may be reproduced in any form by any means, electronic or mechanical, including photocopying, recording, information browsing, storage, or any retrieval system, without specific written permission from the publisher.

ISBNs
978-1-7383082-6-2   (Paperback)
978-1-7383082-7-9   (eBook)

Life
Education
Science
Government

Contents

Endorsements 1
Dedication 6
Introduction 6
Chapter 1: Why "God's" 7
Chapter 2: Why "Given" 9
Chapter 3: Why "Reasons" 11
Chapter 4: Why "Gratitude" 13
Chapter 5: Why "Praise" 15
Chapter 6: Why "Joy" 17
Chapter 7: Scriptures Re: God and Satan 19
Chapter 8: Making Modern Disciples 21
Chapter 9: Objections and Conclusions 23
Index 27
Acknowledgements 29

Dedication

To the triune God of our Western nations who, through His enormous, verifiable, undeniable, superintelligent, loving care and work, earns 100% of the credit for producing all our grown foods and all living cells and entities, including us.

Without our Creator, there would be no food and no Life.

Introduction

As a new believer in 1987, coming from a background in research, engineering, manufacturing, and construction, my first major question was "How does this Creator build living things?"

It took 20 years part-time and 17 years full-time research with God's great help, plus input from 20 PhDs, 9 DScs, 3 MDs, 2 MScs, 3 Mathematicians, and 8 Independent Researchers, to develop this God-based life science. It is a logical replacement for Darwinism's mindless evolution and is based on undeniable and verifiable evidence.

This science is formally called "Atomic Biology" and affectionately nicknamed "God's Biology."

We provide understandable details of His enormous works, love, and care for each one of us every second of every day.

Hopefully, this will inspire your gratitude, praise, and joy in knowing these details of how immensely you are loved and cared for by your superintelligent Creator.   – Tom Rogers

Chapter 1: **Why "God's"?**

With verifiable and undeniable evidence, we now know for certain that "WITHOUT OUR CREATOR, THE GOD OF OUR WESTERN NATIONS, THERE WOULD BE NO FOOD AND NO LIFE."

How do we know this for certain? Because even with all our vast scientific knowledge and highly sophisticated equipment, our scientists cannot come anywhere close to producing even one living cell from elements. **We do not have enough intelligence, and by definition, Darwinisms have no intelligence to use.**

Some big science labs can make copies of a few tiny pieces of a living cell and transplant them into other living cells, but this is many miles away from making a living carrot cell out of dirt.

In 2016, the three Nobel Prize Winners in Chemistry won that prize for making a few simple molecular machines out of atoms. They had worked for thirty-three years to make these little non-living units that needed to be stimulated with ultraviolet light, or an equivalent, to make them move. These are almost infinitely simpler than the simplest of the forty different molecular machines made for our living cells every day of the week.

This is how we know for certain that superintelligence, far above mankind's level, is essential to make all living cells and us.

There is only one such superintelligent entity known to mankind and that is our constant, caring Creator, the triune God of our Western nations.

What do we mean by "the triune God of our Western nations"? We mean the Biblical three-in-one God (the Holy Trinity combo of Father, Son, and Holy Spirit) who is highly recognized by our Governments in the USA, UK, Canada, Australia, and more. They all recognize our God with the national holidays of Christmas, Easter, and Thanksgiving Day, in our justice systems, constitutions, pledges of allegiance, declarations, on our currencies, public buildings, war memorials, and more, with slight variations nation to nation.

This gives all our students the inalienable right to be taught "Why God is so highly recognized by their Government."

The time has come to declare that "THE THEORY OF EVOLUTION IS NOW FACTUALLY FALSIFIED AND MUST BE SENT TO THE HISTORY DEPARTMENT IF TRUTH IS TO BE TAUGHT."

There is no universal common ancestor and there is no construction of living cells without enormous, superintelligent and carefully precise assembly work with atoms.

For over six decades, subtle Satan has been allowed to use Darwin's evolution as a powerful ploy to separate students from their Creator. This has had tragic consequences beyond measure to our students who become adults without the encouraging knowledge that they have a caring and loving Creator.

He is constantly at work making our foods and also constantly at work within each of us building and maintaining our cells and replacing worn-out ones by the millions every second.

In fact, it was the discovery of this enormous work of just replacing our worn-out red blood cells that flipped my part-time curiosity to full-time research and development in 2007. That was when I found that all our red blood cells have to be replaced in about 120 days. Research from C.J.Pallister showed that a 150 pound male receives about 2.3 million new red blood cells every second, 24/7. Then from G.J.Tortora, I found that each red blood cell needs about 280 million molecules of hemoglobin made for it. Then I found from Max Perutz that each molecule of hemoglobin is made of about 10,000 correctly selected and assembled atoms. If you do the math, you will find that a 150 pounder receives about 6400 quadrillion correct atoms made into red blood cells every second of every day.

Put your weight in pounds over 150 and multiply times 6,400,000,000,000,000,000 then give a BIG "Thank you, Lord!"

Chapter 2: Why "Given"?

We are just beginning to count the blessings our Creator, the God of our Western nations, provides for each of us, no charge.

At the end of the last chapter, you were given an idea of the mind-boggling numbers of atoms that God faithfully and reliably sorts, selects, counts, and precisely assembles just to make our replacement red blood cells every second of every day.

But even that humongous number of correct atoms, is less than half. This is because in each same second, He has to be working very hard with a greater number of atoms in the soil of gardens, fields, and orchards, to build our foods for each future second's supply of atoms for new red blood cells. Those foods have roots and peelings we are going to throw away.

To give you an idea of the precision of the work involved in making those each of those 280 million molecules of hemoglobin for each of our red blood cells, the American Red Cross says this: the chemical formula is $C_{2952}H_{4664}N_{812}O_{882}S_8Fe_4$ per molecule.

And this is only one type of cell for our life out of over 200 different types of cells God builds, sustains, and maintains for each one of us.

Now, we get it that these numbers can be a bit overwhelming. We just want you to have some clear and verifiable knowledge regarding the enormous amount of work, care, and love that your Creator provides for you, for each member of your family, and each of your friends, every second of every day.

Perhaps this will give you more reasons to be grateful, to praise God, and to experience some new joy in knowing just how much He cares for each one of us every second of every day.

You may want to thank Him at every mealtime. He earns that and deserves it.

The reason we say "Given" is that God makes no charge for building all our foods and then making, sustaining, and maintaining all our cells and us out of our foods.

It is true that the farmers, and the truckers, and the grocery people have to get paid but God does not. He does all these enormous works and so much more, out of His great love and care for each one of us.

The Bible warns us about false teachings coming at the End of the Age, in several verses including:
"Watch out for false prophets." Matthew 7:15 NIV
How many scammers contact you in a month?
"At that time many will turn away from the faith and will betray and hate each other, and many false prophets will appear and deceive many people." Matthew 24: 10,11 NIV
In the last six decades, how many students have been taught that evolution is the cause of life so they don't need a god.
"But there were also false prophets among the people, just as there will be false teachers among you. They will secretly introduce destructive heresies, even denying the sovereign Lord ...." 2 Peter 2:1 NIV

See the next chapter for the sudden point where this became very widespread.
The teaching of Darwinisms and evolution as the origin and cause of life has misled millions of students into losing their souls since that time.

Our goal is to end this false teaching about life itself. We need believers to learn how much our Creator cares for every person every second of every day.

And then, please share this message, give booklet(s), see our website for ways to help replace the false teaching of Darwinisms and evolution and replace them with the Truth of "God's Biology.".

Chapter 3: **Why "Reasons"?**

When our Western nations were founded, many of our founding fathers understood more clearly, the great work, care and advice that our Creator provides constantly. This is probably because a far larger percentage of the citizens were involved in agriculture and were more aware of the constantly reliable work required to make their food and cattle out of the good earth.

In general, they had the good common sense to understand that all their foods, crops, and cattle did not "just happen" with no intelligent help. Also, more of them paid attention to the great advice for life that is in the Bible, and they were not misled by the false teachings regarding the origin and cause of life. God was given 100% of the credit for food and life by a far greater portion of the people.

We recognize that for the last six decades, our Western nations have been **forcibly deceived** by what we now clearly see as SUBTLE SATAN'S POWERFUL PLOY: TEACHING DARWINISMS EXCLUSIVELY AS THE ORIGIN AND CAUSE OF LIFE TO SEPARATE OUR STUDENTS FROM THEIR CARING CREATOR.

In 1963, Madalyn Murray (O'Hair) and a few atheist friends managed to convince the Supreme Court of the USA to ban the Lord's Prayer and Bible reading from public education.

The negative results from this change were immediate and destructive. Morality took a dive followed immediately by increased drug abuse, unwanted pregnancies, derelict dads, more sexually transmitted diseases, increased health costs, increased policing costs, anxiety, depression, overdoses, and suicides.

These are still increasing major problems today.

For six decades, we have missed the advice in Ephesians. 4:27 "….do not give the devil a foothold." NIV

BRINGING OUR CREATOR BACK TO OUR STUDENTS IS NEEDED TO RESTORE TRUTH FOR LIFE EDUCATION.

The best, truthful, God-based life science is needed to give students and everyone a trustworthy knowledge of the enormous works and care that their Creator provides to each of us. We are proposing our God-based life science of "Atomic Biology" (God's Biology) as a logical science to replace the factually falsified teachings of Darwinisms.

At least until Darwinisms are replaced, let's use "God's Biology" as a sensible supplement in Churches, Christian Schools, Homeschools, and any other institutions seeking to teach Truth for Life. There will no doubt be objections in public schools to any God-based life science in spite of the fact that God is so highly recognized by our Governments.

We have kept our "God's Biology" booklets short and simple in order to make teaching easy. It provides awareness of the enormous works, love, and care that our Creator, the triune God of our Western nations, performs for every person every second of every day.

Chapter 4: Why "Gratitude"?

It is probably true that the vast majority of people have been given no clue about the enormous works and care that God provides for every one of us every second of every day. This is because the educators who control the curricula of life sciences, have purposefully prevented the teaching of any credit for the origin and cause of life, other than to Darwinisms.

To quote one evolutionary professor, Richard Lewontin of Harvard University, "…. *Materialism* (evolution) *is absolute, for we cannot allow a Divine Foot in the door."* [1]

This is both anti-God and anti-science as it disallows scientists from their use of the basic principle for scientific research: "Follow the evidence wherever it leads."

But now we know that materialism and Darwin's Theory of Evolution are **factually falsified**, and our Creator earns 100% of the credit for producing, sustaining, and maintaining all life.

So, why should we have gratitude for God's constant works for us?

(1) He is constantly reliable at making all our delicious and nutritious foods from "the dust."
(2) Then He creates, sustains, and maintains our roughly 100 trillion cells from atoms in our foods.
(3) He heals many wounds and repairs many cells when needed.
(4) He can replace our cells when they need replacement.
(5) He keeps our heart working for over 80 years on average.
(6) He designs, builds, and maintains over 200 different types of cells each with up to 40 different complex molecular machines to give us Life.
(7) He answers our prayers in one of four ways (all starting with "D"): Direct, or Delayed, or Different, or Denied. For examples: Often I will be running late to get to a meeting and cannot find my car keys. Then I remember to ask Him, "Lord, you know I am running late here. Would you help me find my keys, please?" and often before I finish the prayer,

He reminds me where I left them. That is a 'Direct' answer. Sometimes, I have prayed for help in a difficult situation, and He will wait until I have exhausted all my own attempts at solution, then He provides an answer just so I know it is from Him and not my own wisdom. That is a 'Delayed' answer. Then, like the young fellow who started going to college and met some other fellows who had nice cars. He prayed for a nice new Mustang. In a while, he managed to get an old Volkswagen, so that prayer answer was 'Different', but he still got wheels. Then there was a young lady who really wanted and prayed for a close relationship with a particular young man. He turned her down. She was heartbroken as her prayer was 'Denied.' But, as it turned out, that guy was involved in criminal activity and she was better off without him. A little later, she did meet a much better mate for her.

(8) Our bodies and minds are so phenomenally complex that it is amazing we do not have some serious health problems all the time. God builds in an immune system to help keep us healthy most of the time. Often we bring on our own health problems by drinking or consuming some things that cause us harm.

(9) When you start studying the complexity of living cells, especially in our own body, and you learn that scientists cannot come close to creating even one living cell from elements, we can have real gratitude for the superintelligence love, and care that our Creator provides for every one of us every second of every day.

(10) It is a good idea to count our blessings often and give thanks for all that God provides to each of us each day.

You know that it is hard to be grateful and depressed at the same time.

[1] Lewontin, R., *Billions and Billions of Demons,* The New York Review of Books, New York, NY, 9 January, 1997.

Chapter 5: Why "Praise"?

As many of us know, there is something uplifting for our soul when we give thanks to God for His many blessings for each one of us.

Just the act of acknowledging His blessings is like celebrating the fact that we are cared for so much. Praising God with music and song as a group is especially enjoyable.

It is understandable that God is also pleased to be recognized for all the marvelous works He performs for every person every second of every day.

If you have kids, isn't it special when they actually thank you for your loving care for them?

It seems that everyone likes to be appreciated for their efforts.

I remember particularly, a gathering of over 50,000 men at a "Promise-Keepers" conference in the Seattle King Dome. When we all sang some songs of praise to God, a cappella, it seemed like what being in Heaven could be ..... really spine-tingling.

My wife was the nurse-in-charge of 17 operating theaters at St. Paul's Hospital in Vancouver, BC. Several of her patients had near-death experiences during their operations and talked to her later about the gorgeous, bright place that they had gone to. Some wished they had not been brought back to life here on Earth.

The Holy Bible which provides so much great advice for Life, makes it clear that it is good for us to gather together to fellowship with each other as special friends. "And let us consider how to stir up one another to love and good works, not neglecting to meet together, as is the habit of some, but encouraging one another…" Hebrews 10:24-25 ESV

"Praise the Lord! For it is good to sing praises to our God; for it is pleasant and a song of praise is fitting." Psalms 147:1 ESV

"Give thanks to the Lord for He is good. His love endures forever." Psalms 136:1   NIV

Again for emphasis:

WITHOUT THE ENORMOUS LOVE, CARE, AND SUPER-INTELLIGENT WORKS OF OUR CREATOR, THERE WOULD BE NO FOOD AND NO LIFE.

This knowledge alone is good reason for gratitude and to sing praises to Him.

Counting our blessings before going to sleep, is another form of praise that He likes to hear.

A large part of our goal with this life science is to reduce some of the depression and anxiety in the world. Hopefully, by providing solid reasons for virtually everyone to understand how much they are loved and cared for by their Creator, any concern that no one loves them will be unnecessary.

Chapter 6: **Why "Joy?"**

Knowing that superintelligence, enormous work, and constant care are essential for the life of each one of us, including the creating of all our foods and using those foods to create, sustain, and maintain us with all our marvelous parts, are more than abundant reasons for "joy." It is all about His showing of His immense love for each one of us, all the time.

There is so much more to say about His brilliant design and creation work, and His food production, and maintenance for each one of us, that we can rejoice for the many blessings we receive every second of every day.

We have hardly started to list the marvelous gifts that the vast majority of us are given. These grand gifts include eyesight, hearing, tasting, touching, and so many more that we can easily take for granted because His provisions are so constant and reliable here in our Western nations.

It is true that many parts of the world do not have the same abundance that we have and this is why God teaches us to love our neighbors who are in need. He also prompts some of us to be missionaries and all of us to be His disciples.

Some of the great advice in the Bible helps us experience joy.

Also, when in need of something, Jesus teaches us to ASK for what we need. "Ask, and it will be given to you; seek, and you will find; knock, and the door will be open to you. For everyone who asks receives, and the one who seeks finds, and to the one who knocks it will be opened." Matthew 7:7-8 ESV

"Until now you have asked nothing in my name. Ask, and you will receive, that your joy may be full." John 16:24 ESV

The apostle, Paul, tells us about learning "the secret of contentment in all situations." Phillipians 4:11-13 ESV

At our home, we like to thank God for His blessings at every mealtime.

If we will diligently seek "joy," we can find it in abundance especially through counting our blessings.

I remember a great old song with these words:
> "If you're worried and you can't sleep
> Then count your blessings instead of sheep
> And you'll fall asleep counting your blessings."

The Bible has so much great advice for each one of us, especially for dealing with the problems that can come upon us while we are on this Earth. Even the ones we bring upon ourselves, but we have to take some action to help ourselves. Sometimes it just takes a change of attitude.

As the apostle Paul tells us, "I have learned the secret of being content in any and every situation, whether well fed or hungry, whether living in plenty or in want. I can do everything through Him who gives me strength." Phillipians 4:12,13. NIV

I remember an interview that Oprah Winfrey had, where she was asked about some of the mistakes she had made. Her response was that yes, she had made some mistakes but then she would focus on making "the next right move."

Share good clean humor whenever appropriate.
Accentuate your positives as much as possible.
Look for ways for good clean fun.
Remember "Do not grieve, for the joy of (knowing) the Lord is your strength." Nehemiah 8:10 NIV

Chapter 7: Scriptures Re: God and Satan

Scriptures On God's Creative Works For Us (NIV)
 The God we refer to is the triune God of our Western nations (USA, UK, Canada, Australia, and more). He gives no mention of evolution or theistic evolution contributing in any way to the creation or reproduction of any living entities.
 Think of Him when you enter the grocery store and see the apples, oranges, potatoes and carrots, etc. that He has made for your life.
 Without His created foods, we would not exist.

Genesis 1:21 So God created the great creatures of the sea, and every living and moving thing with which the water teems and that moves about in it, according to their kinds, and every winged bird according to its kind. And God saw that it was good.
Genesis 1:26 Then God said, "Let us make mankind in our image, in our likeness, and let them rule over the fish of the sea and the birds in the sky, over the livestock and all the wild animals, and over all the creatures that move along the ground."
Genesis 1:27 So God created mankind in his own image, in the image of God he created them; male and female he created them.
Genesis 2:7 The Lord God formed the man from the dust of the ground and breathed into his nostrils the breath of life, and the man became a living being.
Genesis 2:22 Then the Lord God made a woman from the rib he had taken out of the man, and he brought her to the man.
Psalm 139: 13-14 For you created my inmost being; you knit me together in my mother's womb. I praise you because I am fearfully and wonderfully made;
Ecclesiastes 3:11 He has made everything beautiful in its time.
Isaiah 40:28 Do you not know? Have you not heard? The Lord is the everlasting God, the Creator of the ends of the earth. He will not grow tired or weary, and his understanding no one can fathom.
Romans 1:20 For since the creation of the world, God's invisible qualities -- his eternal power and divine nature---have been clearly seen, being understood from what has been made, so that people are without excuse.

Romans 11:36 For from Him and through Him and for Him are all things. To Him be the glory forever! Amen

Ephesians 2:10 For <u>we are God's handiwork</u>, created in Christ Jesus to do good works, which God prepared in advance for us to do.

Scriptures On Satan's Destructive Deeds (NIV)

Mark 1:13 ... and he (Jesus) was in the desert forty days, being tempted by Satan.

Luke 13:16 "Then should not this woman ... whom Satan has bound for eighteen long years, be set free on the Sabbath day?

Luke 22:3 Then Satan entered Judas, called Iscariot, one of the Twelve. (Inspiring betrayal of Jesus).

Acts 10:38 ...how God anointed Jesus of Nazareth with the Holy Spirit and power, and how He went around doing good and healing all who were under the power of the devil, because God was with Him.

Romans 16:20 The God of peace will soon crush Satan under your feet.

2 Corinthian 11:3 But I am afraid that just as Eve was deceived by the serpent's cunning, your minds may somehow be led astray from your sincere and pure devotion to Christ.

2 Corinthians 11:14 And no wonder, for Satan himself masquerades as an angel of light.

Ephesians 4:27 ... and do not give the devil a foothold.

1 Timothy 1:20 Among them are Hymenaeus and Alexander, whom I have handed over to Satan to be taught not to blaspheme.

James 4:7 Submit yourselves, then, to God. Resist the devil, and he will flee from you.

1 Peter 5:8 Be alert and of sober mind. Your enemy, the devil, prowls around like a roaring lion looking for someone to devour.

Chapter 8: **Making Modern Disciples**

The Greatest Commandment

"Love the Lord your God with all your heart and with all your soul and with all your mind. This is the first and greatest commandment. And the second is like it: 'Love your neighbor as yourself.' All the Law and the Prophets hang on these two commandments." Matthew 22:37-40 NIV

The Great Commission

"Therefore, go and make disciples of all nations, baptizing them in the name of the Father, and of the Son, and of the Holy Spirit ...." Matthew 28:19 NIV

Keep these two pieces of advice in mind as you work and look after your family and play. There is joy in living within God's will for your life. Ask, seek, and knock to determine His will for you at the beginning of each day.

Equipping Modern Disciples

In Jesus days on Earth, He performed many "miracles," the climax of which was His resurrection from the dead to defeat death.

He raised several others from their dead state as well as making the blind to see, the lame to walk, the leper to heal, the demon- possessed to be free, and believers to be saved, as He still does today.

Some may say, "God doesn't do 'miracles' today," but now you can point out your new knowledge of some verifiable and undeniable "Facts of Life":

1. God makes each one of us out of dirt with His 'miraculous' two-step creative works, i.e. (1) He makes our foods out of atoms in the dirt, then (2) He makes all our living cells out of atoms from our foods.

2. He replaces our worn-out red blood cells at a rate of over 2,000,000 per second, each one of which is created with about 280,000,000 molecules of hemoglobin and of these, each molecule is being made out of almost 10,000 correct atoms from our foods. (Formula: $C_{2952}H_{4664}N_{812}O_{882}S_8Fe_4$ according to The American Red Cross).
3. For the number of correct atoms per second being made into red blood cells to replace our worn-out ones, as we speak, do the math and ask, "Is this perhaps a bit 'miraculous'?"
4. The DNA molecules made for about 80 trillion of our living cells, also have to be constructed out of atoms from our foods. For each of these DNA molecules for each of these cells, about 3 billion pairs of bases have to be precisely arranged to help manage the activities of 200 different types of cells each having up to 40 different, complex molecular machines. (Another bit of a 'miracle'?)
5. Each of the four different types of bases are not terribly complex but the precision required for the assembly of each one is a bit startling to me:
   <u>A</u>denine - chemical formula $C_5 H_5 N_5$
   <u>G</u>uanine -   "   " $C_5 H_5 N_5 O_1$
   <u>C</u>ytosine -   "   " $C_4 H_5 N_3 O_1$
   <u>T</u>hymine -   "   " $C_5 H_6 N_2 O_2$

   Notice how similar the formulae are for these bases. As each one is being constructed for us using atoms from our digestive system via our bloodstreams, it is critical that the builder be absolutely precise in the selection, counting, and placement of the correct numbers of the required atoms, as well as fastening the 6,000,000,000 right bases into correct pairs then placing each pair in the proper sequences in programming our DNA for the various required functions in each of our cells. What great intelligence, love and care this requires.
6. You might say that every living cell and entity is a bit of a miracle, as mankind has nowhere near enough intelligence to build even the simplest living cell out of atoms.
7. Then there are the four types of prayer answers: 'Direct,' 'Delayed,' 'Different,' and 'Denied' but replaced with better.

Chapter 9: Objections and Conclusions

Of course, there will be loud objections from atheists and evolutionists against replacing Darwinisms with a God-based life science because it upsets their worldview.

We will hear, "There is separation of church and state, you know. This 'Atomic Biology' is just religion in disguise!"

Answer: "Yes, the intended concept of the church not telling the state what to do and the state not telling the church what to do, is a good one. But if you want to understand how your foods are reliably and constantly made out of dirt and how all of your complex cells are made out of your foods, you will need some truthful life science. This permanent job of making your foods and making your cells takes enormous, highly complex scientific work every second of every day. So if you want truth rather than fiction, listen up. The forefathers of our Western nations understood a lot of this by intuition and common sense. Hopefully, there is still some of that around. They also appreciated the worker who was doing the work of making food and life out of dirt. Certainly, no church can do that. And as has been proven over the last seventy years, no scientists can do this either."

This leads us back to our beginnings as Western democracies (USA, UK, Canada, Australia, and more). They knew Who the Creator of their foods and cattle is and they were grateful. This is why they appreciated and highly recognized this wonderful, caring, creator who was doing all this work out of pure love for each person. He does not charge anything for His constant, brilliant, creative works and supply of sustenance and maintenance for everyone.

The governments are obviously not religions but they do show their appreciation by highly recognizing God with the national holidays of Christmas, Easter, and Thanksgiving Day, in our justice systems, declarations, pledges of allegiance, constitutions, on currencies, public buildings, war memorials, and more, with slight variations nation to nation.

And this gives all our students the inalienable right to be taught "Why God is so highly recognized by their government."

We hope that this booklet has given you some great physical reasons for "joy" and for solidifying your faith.

You can share this verifiable and undeniable knowledge of the enormous life-giving works, love, and care that our Creator provides to every person every second of every day and at no charge.

We do have to remember that there is a real enemy who works against us. "Be sober-minded; be watchful. Your adversary the devil prowls around like a roaring lion, seeking someone to devour." 1 Peter 5:8   NIV

It is our firm belief that one of subtle Satan's most powerful ploys has been to deceive those who control biology curricula in public education into enforcing the teaching of evolution-only regarding the origin and cause of life. **This has been used to separate our students from their creator for over six decades.**

But also remember that the Theory of Evolution is now factually falsified because superintelligence is now proven to be essential for building every living cell and entity, including us. By definition, evolution has no intelligence to use. **This is why Darwinisms are factually falsified regarding both the origin and the cause of life.**

WITHOUT OUR CREATOR, THE GOD OF OUR WESTERN NATIONS, THERE WOULD BE NO FOOD AND NO LIFE.

We hope you agree that the use of Darwinisms to separate our students from their Creator must be stopped. The loss of souls, the rising crime, hardships, health-care costs and policing costs can all be reduced by bringing this Truth for Life Education back to our students.

We have the God-based life science called "Atomic Biology" and nicknamed "God's Biology" to replace the factually falsified Darwinisms with "Truth For Life Education."

Those teachers and professors who are forced to continue teaching Darwinisms are being forced to lie to their students about life itself.

What conscientious teacher or professor really wants their legacy to be that they continued to lie to their students when Truth was available?

Your participation can be historic in this overdue solution to the devastating ploy of separating students from their Creator. The truth will soon win if many of us help to spread this vital news. We have customizable booklets and textbooks, speakers, and are asking boldly for publicity funds and angel partnerships.

Each part of this will help to bring the God of our nations back to our students.

Please pray and participate in this historic advancement for the better life of our citizens.

www.GodsBiology.com

Index

Atoms 3,6-9,12,21,22
Blessings 9,14,15,17,18
Cells 6-9,13,14,21
Church 21,23
Conclusions 23
Devil 12,20,24
Disciples 17,21
Education 4,9,11,20,22-25, 29
Factually falsified 8,12,13, 24, 25
Hemoglobin 8,9,22
God 1-25
Government 7,8,23
Gratitude 6,13,14,29
Inalienable 8,24
Jesus 7,17,20,21
Joy 6,9,17,18,21,24
Lewontin, Richard 13
Lord 8,11,13,15,18-20
Lord's Prayer 10
Nations 7,9,11,17,19,21, 23-25

Objections 23
Pallister, C.J. 8
Perutz, Max 8
Praise 8,12
Project 17,29
Quadrillion 8
Red blood cells 8,9,22
Satan 8,11,19,20,24
Scriptures 19,20
Separation 14
State 14
Tortora, G.J. 8
Triune 6,7,19
Truth ,12,23-25,29
Undeniable 6,7,21,24
Verifiable 6,7,9,21,24

Acknowledgments

It is with great appreciation that we thank those who have helped to bring this "Truth For Life Education Project" to this point. First and foremost is my wonderful wife, Bonnie, who has helped in the research and development of this God-based life science for two decades along with my techie son, Derek. Next are my great co-authors, Dr. Graham McLennan and Dr. Jerry Bergman, my special coach, Norman Wright, my editor, David V. Bassett, and my fund-raising helper, Suzanne Diamond.

Then, of course, are the 45 scholars who provided input for the development of the God-based life science of Atomic Biology, which is affectionately nicknamed "God's Biology."

Then there are the many special encouragers who helped to inspire the continuation of this project of bringing our awesome Creator back to students and citizens, in spite of the strong opposition to God's Truth.

With appreciation and gratitude, we thank all who have helped and continue to help make this God-based life science and "Truth For Life Education Project" a blessing for everyone.

Other Books in the "Darwin's Replacement Series":
"God's Biology – Darwin's Replacement (Textbook)
"God Is In The Grocery Store" (Summary for Everyone)
"How We Are Amazingly Made" (Summary Introduction)

HELP US MAKE THIS WORLD A BETTER PLACE!

Contact Us

www.GodsBiology.com or www.atomicbiology.com

www.ingramcontent.com/pod-product-compliance
Lightning Source LLC
Chambersburg PA
CBHW042318090526
44583CB00024BA/3113